TMJ and Parkinson's Disease

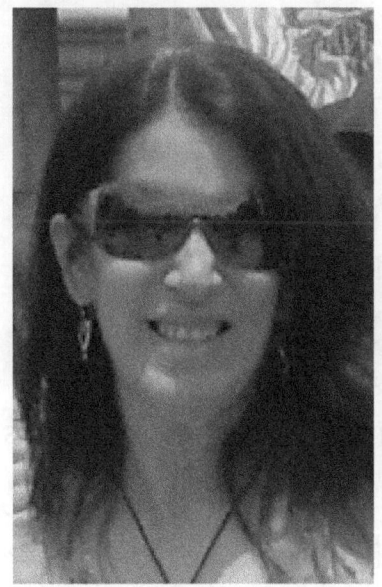

TMJ Adjustments
and
Parkinson's
Disease

Tell us about the time when you were first diagnosed with Parkinson's

CHERYL: It started out when I was 42 years old. About a year after my first child was born I first noticed that I couldn't swing my arm when I was walking. Then I noticed that I really wasn't washing my hair with my left hand when I was taking showers. All of these things started slowly, gradually getting worse. Other things started coming up and I thought,

© Parkinsons Recovery   1

TMJ and Parkinson's Disease

"That's odd!"

I went to a doctor. They sent me to a neurologist and the neurologist did a slew of tests, speculating there might be a brain tumor or a lot of other different possibilities. To make a long story short, it took about two years for a diagnosis of Parkinson's to come because there was no Parkinson's history in my family and I was so young. Two years later I was diagnosed with Parkinson's and I thought, "I can beat this thing, I can do this, I'm going to try anything holistic that I can try" Because I'm kind of an anti-medication person, I never even took an aspirin in my life. I just didn't get headaches. I never got sick at work. I just couldn't believe that I had Parkinson's

I thought, okay I'm going to go to a chiropractor. I went to a chiropractor. I went to an acupuncturist. I went to a Chinese herbalist. I would try these therapies for a good six, eight months

TMJ and Parkinson's Disease

giving them what I thought was a long time to take effect. I understand that holistic medicine takes a while to incorporate into your body. I did the hyperbaric chamber which actually did me a little bit of benefit.

I tried a lot of different therapies and I was just getting worse. I just couldn't stop it and I had to admit it and I had to get help. I needed to get on the medication and I did not want to get on the medication because I read about all the side effects. It was just horrible for me to have to do this but I was between a rock and a hard place and medication was the last resort.

I have been on the meds now for I think about five or six years and I take the pretty standard regime of Requip, Amantadine, Sinemet - the standard protocol for this disease. I think everybody gets to all those different meds at some point or a reasonable facsimile

TMJ and Parkinson's Disease

thereof. I'm still thinking and I'm still hoping, I had hoped that there's something else that can get me out of this because I know it's not going to come from the medical community. I know the only thing that they're thinking about is drugs, more drugs and more drugs and brain surgery and those aren't very good options for me; I don't like either of them.

I remember going to Parkinson's support groups and they would have guest speakers come in. Some of these speakers would be therapists. They would tell you, you have to learn to accept your disease and you have to learn to accept your life the way it is. Grow from there. Develop from there. Learn new skills. I would raise my hand and say, "I will never accept this disease." I'm looking at this guy, like he's got four eyes; it's like, "Are you nuts? I want my life back! I really do, I want my life back and to tell me to accept it is not helping me, just tell me how to get out of this!" That's just my mindset about this whole thing.

I just knew there had to be a way out of it and I just have never stopped looking, but at the same token I'm a realist and I'm not going to not take the drugs. I've got two small children who are actually ages ten and seven right now. They're my world and I've got to keep up with them. One of them is a boy and he's a very active little boy. Sometimes I just want to lie down but I can't. It's more than a full time job; it's developing two lives. As far as the Parkinson's, I didn't get blessed but as far as having those kids I did. God gave me a gift in spite of all of this trauma.

Did you see an improvement in your symptoms when you took prescription medicines?

CHERYL: Absolutely; the drugs masked over a lot of the symptoms but I still felt this current going through my body. As much as I was able to physically do things I just never felt normal. The way the

TMJ and Parkinson's Disease

drugs would affect me is like a wave washing over my body – one minute I wasn't normal. The next minute I was.

I've gotten a lot of side-effects from the drugs. I've got dyskinesia. I've got dystonia in my feet, I've got dyskinesia in my upper limbs. I've gotten a slew of other side-effects that I don't need to go into, but those are the two big ones. The side-effects are real and they're uncomfortable, almost more uncomfortable than the disease for me. I couldn't read my own handwriting and I love to write. I've got a pen collection. I've been writing for years and to lose my penmanship for me personally was just horrific. My facial mask, I could feel when I would smile because my face was just so blank. I couldn't walk with certain shoes on because they would just flop off my feet. Just a slew of things were going wrong for me. I couldn't put a sandwich in a zip-lock baggie; I couldn't make that motion. I couldn't stuff an envelope - just that

TMJ and Parkinson's Disease

pushing motion, my hand wouldn't do that. I couldn't fold laundry. I couldn't, I couldn't, I couldn't. It was just a lot of different things that I was losing the battle to. Yes, there were a lot of symptoms that were affecting my life.

> **Tell us what has happened recently to turn your situation around**

CHERYL: A month ago I went to a support group, and a dentist came into the support group. He was very clear. He said there are about 50 dentists around the country do what he does. He's a TMJ expert and works specifically with movement disorder patients. He's a member of the American Academy of Cranial Facial Pain. He said, "I'm not going to tell you I can cure Parkinson's. I don't know anything about Parkinson's. But I can tell you I can make you symptom-free, so if that's the cure, that's what I can do. You will be symptom-free after you're done with my device".

TMJ and Parkinson's Disease

I thought to myself, "Right." Who is this guy? There was a group of us at the meeting that included a woman that I've known for the past three years. She's always been in some form of a wheel chair, walker, or a cane with four prongs on the bottom. Her husband is always with her assisting her. He is a very kind gentleman, always helping his wife out, but she could not move around by herself. She needed some form of assistance.

The dentist said to this lady, "You young lady, come up here." She was using her cane this particular night and walked up to the dentist. He placed a tongue depressor in her mouth sideways. He said, "What I'm doing is, there's a little bone right where your upper and your lower jaw meet. It's about the size of a cat's claw. It's your temporal mandela mandible (temporo-mandibular). It is a little bone right next to your carotid artery, right where your upper and lower jaw meet. He then said, "I'm adjusting that bone, I'm shifting that bone, because when that bone is out of alignment all kinds of symptoms occur. When that bone is adjusted and in proper alignment your symptoms will go away." That's basically the long and the short of his presentation.

He placed this tongue depressor in her mouth. He grabbed her cane and he said, "Now go walk down the hallway." She stands there momentarily and she grabs her cane back. It was a little brash, but he wanted to prove a point. He goes, "Now go walk down the hallway" and he grabs the cane. She stands there momentarily. She is just standing there. He said again, "Walk down the hallway." So, she takes a step and she starts walking down this hallway. She's walking. She comes back down the hallway and then she's walking around the room and she's smiling and she does not want to stop walking. She can't believe she's walking. I'm looking at her and I can't believe she's walking. If did

TMJ and Parkinson's Disease

not know her I would think this was a plant.

It was too unbelievable. It was like watching a miracle. If there are any miracles, this was a miracle because I've known this lady for three years and she cannot do that. She's got a tongue depressor in her mouth and she's walking. It was fantastic! That caught my attention.

I see her about three weeks to a month later at a Parkinson's fund raiser. She is dancing wither husband. She is dancing! This woman was in a wheelchair before. She went to this dentist obviously because she saw the benefit. Now I'm seeing her again and she's dancing with her husband. I was floored. I mean if I believed when I saw it the first time I really believed what I saw the second time. I thought to myself, "I've got to try this! I've got to try this!"

There was another gentleman at the fundraiser who was also at the support group meeting. He went and got himself an appliance as well. I saw him at the fundraiser and he was carrying back four glasses of wine back to the table he was sitting at. There is no way this gentleman could even have walked back to his table nevertheless carry four glasses of wine without spilling them and walking back to the table. It was unbelievable. They both had a appliance in their mouth. I thought, "I want some of that! I want some of that good health!"

But I was scared. I was really scared. I mean what if it doesn't work for me? I'm not in a wheelchair yet. I'm not doing great but I'm not in a wheelchair yet. What if it doesn't work for me? It's a lot of money, it's scary. But at the same time there are no side-effects, I'm not popping pills. There is no brain surgery involved. It is not invasive. It is not cutting into me. It is like you are wearing a retainer in your mouth and I thought to myself, "I've got to do this. I've got to do this. I can't deny what I'm seeing."

I talked to my neurologist, I called him up and of course he said, "You're wasting your money. You are wasting your time. I couldn't find anything on the internet about it. Nobody else had heard about it." My doctor is a great guy. He is at the cutting edge and at the UCLA Medical Center. I really going to a movement disorder specialist and not seeing a local neurologist in my community. I'm really at where I think is the cutting edge of professional health for the Parkinson's community because I'm a young onset patient and I wanted to get the best of the best. He said, try it if you have to, but don't spend a lot of money. He was trying to be positive with me but at the same token he doesn't believe that anything's really going to come of this. So, I did because I had to, because it's just my nature, because I know what I saw and I know what state Sally was in and the other gentleman was in. I couldn't deny

TMJ and Parkinson's Disease

what I saw.

So I went to this dentist and I got myself an appliance. The first day Robert, the first day, I was folding laundry at night. There is no way when I'm off meds at night that I can fold laundry and I just did it.

I called this appliance "Henry". I've nick-named it because it sounds like I have a toaster in my mouth if I just keep calling it an appliance. I don't have a toaster in my mouth so, it's Henry. And Henry just works in miraculous ways. It is very slow. It is very gradual. When I say slow, I don't mean slow like it's slow in healing. It just kind of catches you off guard. All of the sudden you are doing something that your body had forgotten how to do and you're just doing it. So many things I've realized that I'm doing right now and so many things I don't realize that other people are pointing out to me that I'm doing, like the other morning I just

TMJ and Parkinson's Disease

hopped out of bed. I don't know how many Parkinson's patients hop out of bed but I sure didn't. You just don't hop out of bed. You pull yourself up, you roll over as best you can, you kind of fall out of bed. I'm hopping out of bed now. So many things have changed in my life since I've gotten Henry. I can't even begin to tell you.

Are you wearing Henry right now?

Yes I am.

Can people tell that you have an appliance in your mouth?

CHERYL: No. You would not notice it, but to me it feels like there's a table in my mouth. I'm not going to tell you it's comfortable. I'm getting used to it but it does feel awkward. I mean, you have this retainer in your mouth. I've never had braces before as a child or anything so I've never really experienced having anything in my mouth before like this. I wear Henry all day long and I have a separate

TMJ and Parkinson's Disease

piece that I wear in the evening, a night retainer. They are both specially made.

This dentist has all this special equipment. It takes about 3 hours to get tested. He does a series of different tests. He does TMJ tests. He does Head X-rays. He measures the width of your mouth and the length. He looks at all kinds of things before he actually makes this appliance. They are all individually custom made depending on your level of what you need.

Does the appliance have to be adjusted periodically by the dentist?

CHERYL: I go back once a week and get it adjusted, yes. It's an ongoing process with the dentist, you keep getting it adjusted but that's fine because every time he adjusts it, he's just tightening it so it stays in your mouth better and it feels better in your mouth and when he adjusts it I think the benefits come out a little bit more. I can tell you on the first day I noticed that I was folding laundry. That

TMJ and Parkinson's Disease

was I thought, fantastic. The second day I was putting my pants on and I was like, "Oh my God, I just put my pants on! I can't believe it!" I went to brush my teeth and I didn't go for the electric toothbrush I just went for my manual toothbrush. "I can brush my teeth!" Things just start happening and if you're aware of it you can quantify it and tell people about it. I'm putting sandwiches in the zip-lock baggies.

There's so many little things that are coming back into my life that weren't in my life before that I was losing a grip on and it's the first time that I've ever seen this happen. I mean I've been taking medications for five, six years now and now I'm able to do these things. As a matter of fact I'm going at four hours now in between medications and I'm slowly starting to reduce my medication. My goal is to be symptom-free but the process is just amazing to me. It's like you have an infection on your arm and the infection

TMJ and Parkinson's Disease

won't go away and it's just there for the longest time and all of the sudden you start seeing the infection around your arm starting to heal and you see the edges healing and that's the stage I'm in right now. I'm one month into this appliance. The dentist says that I'm going to wear it for about six or seven months and at that point I should be able to take it off and I was like, "Oh my God, could that really be true? Could that really be true?" I didn't want to tell too many people about the appliance because I'm still waiting for the shoe to drop.

So I'm in the dentist office the other day and I'm getting my check up and I see a gentleman who had started the appliance before I did. He was in the dentist's office the same time I was, and I said, "How are you feeling?" He says, "A thousand times better." I said, "A thousand times better?" He says, "I'm completely symptom free!" And I just said, "Oh my God!" He says, "I'm normal Cheryl. I'm normal. I

TMJ and Parkinson's Disease

couldn't swing a golf club seven months ago; I just played 18 holes of golf yesterday."

I'm thinking to myself, I know how good I'm doing, and this just encouraged me to just come out with it because it is real and it is working and it is going to keep getting better and better for me too. I just thought, this can't be a secret. This is real. This is helping. This is the first time in ten years that I've seen my symptoms reversing and that's just too huge not to tell people about. It's just phenomenal.

I'm already feeling it, I'm walking around the room; I couldn't talk to you this quickly or this clearly just a month ago. It would have been impossible.

My energy level is better. My confidence level is better. I actually sold my house and I'm going to start packing up and start moving. Things just start coming to you. I was sitting at the keyboard the other day and my hands went on the home

TMJ and Parkinson's Disease

keys and I just started typing normally and I'm looking at myself going, "Where did that come from?!" It just gradually reclaims – it's just like your body remembers something it forgot it knew how to do and it's just starting to do it again; it's like my body's saying, "Thank you, I'm healing. I'm not medicated, I'm not getting this massive rush of ability; I'm slowly getting my ability back." It's real. It's undeniably, quantifiably, verifiably real.

I went to my neurologist because I was telling him this is really happening, this is real and you've got to tell people about this. And he says, "Cheryl you can't. It's just not going to happen." I said, "Let me come in and you can see me for yourself." This was after like two and a half weeks I went to my neurologist and he said, "I can see an improvement in your walk, and I can see your dystonia is better but I only see you twenty minutes at a time so let's just see how this goes." He had to admit

TMJ and Parkinson's Disease

that he saw an improvement because it is there. But he also kind of took it away because he still doesn't believe it himself. I think what will convince him is if I can reduce my medication and or completely eliminate it which is actually my goal. He says he'll help me do that, so I give him that. That is great. I appreciate that he's doing that, but he's still skeptical.

That's the problem that I'm having is a lot of people say, "Well, let me go ask my doctor about that appliance." I'm trying to tell my friends this is really working and they can see that it's working but people are skeptical about it. There's nothing written up about it. They just had the Parkinson's World Conference meeting in Scotland and all these countries came together to exchange information about Parkinson's disease. All they did was talk about surgery and medication and nobody mentioned this. Nobody even talked about it and you know why? The pharmaceutical companies – and this is

TMJ and Parkinson's Disease

from my doctor who told me this – the pharmaceutical companies control the clinical trials. If it's not pharmaceutical-related then they're not going to pay for the trial because they're not going to make any money off of it. My doctor said that there's no way that anybody's going to put this on the market because without clinical trials the FDA's not going to put it on the market and there's not going to be any clinical trials because nobody can support the clinical trials to do this because it's the pharmaceutical companies that have the money to make these trials. If they're not going to make any money at it they're not going to have a trial, so it's just not going to get out unless it gets out from word of mouth. So I have to be a spokesperson for this thing because this is real and this is really reversing my Parkinson's systems.

It's unbelievable Robert. I can't tell you how much, much, much, much, much better I am in one month and you will feel

TMJ and Parkinson's Disease

it the first day. Sally was walking with a dip stick in her mouth; I mean this thing can't be a secret anymore. It can't be just word of mouth it has to be told via the internet or the radio or TV, you know it just has to get out to the masses and people have to believe that they can get better because they really can. I never gave up hope that it was going to happen.

Have there been any non-motor improvements?

CHERYL: I'm definitely thinking a lot more clearly, I mean a lot more quickly. I just couldn't annunciate myself; I couldn't speak fast enough and get it out quickly enough. I found my voice had softened to a level where I couldn't be heard so I stopped speaking, I stopped taking invitations because I couldn't keep up with people. So you slowly start shrinking out of sight and things like that just start happening gradually and naturally because you're just not the same as everybody; so I think those are non-motor

TMJ and Parkinson's Disease

issues.

> **How do you recommend we find a dentist? Is there a listing somewhere?**

CHERYL: The place to go is the Parkinson's Research Organization and there's a lady named Jo Rosen there and she's got a listing of all these different dentists that are registered, that are a part of the Academy of Cranial Facial Pain. *But there's a small segment of dentists. They're probably mostly in the metropolitan area.*

> **Detail out for us precisely what happened during your initial visit to the dentist.**

CHERYL: When you first go the price is 75 dollars for a consultation, I think that's probably across the board what my dentist charges everybody. He's going to test you and see if you qualify to get an appliance, if he can help you. He's got a series of tests that he makes to see if that's possible. The tests are in-office and innocuous. There's nothing invasive or

TMJ and Parkinson's Disease

anything like that. If he feels that he can help you he discusses with you the therapy and the protocol and what it's going to take for you, because every person is different. For example, if you don't have any teeth he's got to make a special appliance and that's a particularly hard case because the appliance adheres to your teeth. Even if you don't have teeth, if you've had bridge work, your situation is different. Everybody is different so he'll discuss with you what your particular case is like.

If you decide to proceed with the procedure, you come back and the second appointment is about three hours worth of testing. He takes x-rays and his office staff will talk to you about what you have to do to take measurements. After that is all done you come back for a third visit. That is when he actually makes the appliance. It's basically a mold that he takes from an impression from your teeth. The cast takes about a week to ten days to

TMJ and Parkinson's Disease

make. This particular dentist doesn't have an in-office place to make the mold so sends it out to a lab. Then you come back and you get it fitted. The whole process took me about three weeks from start to finish and then I was wearing my appliance.

I thought, oh I'm going to feel something immediately. When I got out of my chair from the dentist's office I didn't feel anything immediately. I thought, okay, we'll just give it some time. We'll see what happens and that first day I did experience the benefit of Henry, as I named my appliance. From then on everyday for the first two weeks there was something new that I was able to do that I couldn't do the day before. When I went to pick up my kid from school, my seven year old said, "Mommy, you're walking so much better today." He didn't know I had been to the dentist and was wearing Henry. He just threw that out there, and so it was visible even to a seven year old that I was

TMJ and Parkinson's Disease

improving.

> **How much does it cost to have this appliance made?**

CHERYL: It varies. It depends on your mouth and what the dentist has to do to get it in there and make it work for you. It costs anywhere between three to twelve thousand dollars. My dentist has a payment plan. If you can't pay the full amount up front, he's got a payment plan that he can put you on for two, three, four, up to five years. When I first heard the price I thought, "Oh my God that's so expensive, three to twelve thousand dollars, oh my God! How am I going to afford that?" Then I thought to myself, you know what, I would mortgage my house if I could get rid of this disease, if I could feel symptom-free. I would give anything, I would pay double that. I started thinking; I've had this for ten years, that's a thousand dollars a year. I've probably paid close to that in less than ten years. This year alone I can't

TMJ and Parkinson's Disease

even tell you what my medical bills are and my medicine bills have been. I've fallen into that donut hole with Medicare with the medication. I think you get like up to 2,500 dollars if you're on Medicare that they'll cover and then you fall into this big donut hole. I've fallen into the donut hole so I'm paying for my medication as it is right now. It's costing me a lot more to stay on the pills and to stay medicated than it is to have Henry. You know that is a fair price to reclaim my health and get my life back.

> ## Can payments be spread out for as long as five years?

CHERYL: Yes. My dentist gave me that option so it would be like two hundred dollars a month over five years or something like that. I thought about going that rout. What if the appliance doesn't work? But it does work and it was worth every penny of it.

TMJ and Parkinson's Disease

Does the initial charge also cover the adjustments that are required?

CHERYL: Yes. That's correct. I guess he saw the look on my face when he told me the price and he said now that includes everything. " I'm not going to nickel and dime you, I'm not going to charge you for every adjustment or every time you need an adjustment and you want to come in, this is one shot and that's all I'm going to charge you." He said, now if you lose your appliance it's going to cost you extra money so don't lose it, because then I have to make another one. Other than that he's not going to charge you anything else.

How long is the treatment period?

CHERYL: Well the person that doesn't have teeth is going a little bit longer because it's a little bit more problematic. A woman without her teeth was quoted a year before she regains her complete health back. I was quoted seven months.

TMJ and Parkinson's Disease

> **Will the time between appointments lengthen over time?**

CHERYL: I assume so, yes.

> **What got you started on this path?**

CHERYL: Parkinsons Resource Organization: www.parkinsonsresource.org The people there are real nice and real friendly as very helpful and they're the ones that got me started on this path. The 800 number is 877-775-4111 and then they have an office number that you can just call directly it's 760-773-5628. The director is Jo Rosen

> **Does your dentist also do general dental work?**

CHERYL: He is a TMJ expert. He noticed that over the 30 years that he's been doing this TMJ work that his patients were talking and telling him, "My headaches are gone, I'm sleeping better, I've regained my balance, and my shaking has stopped." I never really had the problems with the tremors so much personally but these are

TMJ and Parkinson's Disease

the things that his patients were telling him. So they were getting their TMJ work done and so he started connecting the dots and he started looking more into this and that's when he found these other pioneers in this field. So yes, he does more than just Henry, he's a full dentist.

> **Is an internet search useful using the words "TMJ" and "movement disorders"?**

CHERYL: Probably not. It's so new and the word is just now getting out about it. I would like people to know not to have any fear because that fear is the thing that holds most people back from anything in life. Parkinson's is scary. Getting well is scary as well, believe it or not. You can lead a horse to water but you can't make him drink. I don't know why you can't make him drink when the horse is tired and thirsty, you know but people are scared to try this. It's scary because it's a lot of money. It's scary because what if it doesn't work for you? I had all these same fears and I would just really like to

TMJ and Parkinson's Disease

encourage people, don't be afraid of yourself. Don't be afraid to get well. Don't be afraid that you can improve because you really can with this treatment.

I personally know three people that are undergoing it. All three people are if not better, getting better and Jo Rosen has told that she knows of 30 people who have improved. Obviously she's more in the center of things. I'm just in my little world here.

Was your improvement steady?

CHERYL: Henry worked for me for about two weeks and then I felt like I plateaued. I was waiting for 'what am I going to be able to do today?' I thought okay, well this is all I get; I'm still happy, I'm still thrilled and I still got more benefits than I had two weeks ago out of this and then all of the sudden one day it's like Henry woke up again and started working for me again. I talked to a friend who also had an appliance fitted. He said you'll have a

TMJ and Parkinson's Disease

series of ups and downs. I just experienced my first one. You tend to see gradual but rapid improvement and then you plateau. I think your body's just like adjusting to it. Oh my God do you realize everything I've just done? Your body needs a little time to assimilate everything and then it goes to the next level and then it plateaus and then it goes to the next level, and then it plateaus and then it goes to the next level. So if anybody does try this and they experience this plateau, it's part of the process.

> What would want to say to a person who has just been diagnosed with Parkinson's disease?

CHERYL: I would tell them that there's hope. It's not a death sentence. You're lucky you're in the year 2010 and you called me because I can steer you towards something that will save you a lot of time and money and anxiety and maybe if you just try Henry first before you went anyplace else you wouldn't have to go through anything like I did. And they

© *Parkinsons Recovery*   32

TMJ and Parkinson's Disease

couldn't even imagine the magnitude of that; what I went through. You just can't even imagine it. So if I could catch somebody before they went through any of that I would really try and tell them that they can avoid a lot of anxiety and a lot of discomfort and a lot of embarrassment and a lot of being humbled by this disease and they can continue their life; they have a chance now.

Caller 1: **Is there hope for someone who's had Parkinson's for 22 years?**

CHERYL: Of course there is. I don't know what stage you're at but this woman was in a wheelchair and I don't know how long she's had Parkinson's but she got to that stage and she was walking so yes I would say absolutely. I think after 22 years you're probably that much more progressed and it might take maybe, I mean I'm not the doctor, I'm not the dentist, maybe it would take you a little bit longer but I think you'll feel the

TMJ and Parkinson's Disease

benefits of it as quickly as Charlene did.

Caller 2: Does the TMJ appliance move the jaw forward?

CHERYL: That's absolutely what he wants to do is move my jaw forward, open up the airway passages and relieve the pressure. He also wants me to have chiropractic adjustments.

Caller 2: Chiropractic adjustments from a cranial-sacral chiropractor?

CHERYL: Yes.

Caller 2: I thought so. So he's trying to stretch out that digastric muscle. I've heard for a long time that is was the digastrics muscle that needs to be addressed and I had mine worked on but it did not make a difference, so I'm thinking that probably holding the jaw forward for an extended period of time like your appliance does may have an effect that I'm looking for.

CHERYL: That will complete the process,

TMJ and Parkinson's Disease

absolutely; sounds like it.

CHERYL: No, that was just a conversation. The second appointment was just testing to see how I'm biting, how my jaws move, they're testing to see where your bone structure is, they take a full head x-ray, so there's no improvement during the first or second visit, you only get the improvement once the appliance is physically in your mouth.

That would be the third visit. You might try the dip stick thing that he did with that other woman. If you put a dip stick in your mouth or a pencil and you just put it horizontally in your mouth and shove it all the way back you might be able to make an adjustment to your jaw, to that bone and you can swing your arms around; stand with your feet on the ground and swing your arms around and then put that thing in your mouth and

© *Parkinsons Recovery*   35

TMJ and Parkinson's Disease

swing your arms again and see if you get more movement. You should be able to.

> **Caller 4: Were you actually able to reduce your medication level already?**

CHERYL: I have actually stopped taking my last Sinemet pill at night and I take Requip XL two times a day four milligrams each and my second Requip tablet I've reduced to two milligrams. Yes. I have started reducing the medications.

> **Caller 4: Did you have a lot of fatigue with your Parkinson's symptoms before getting your TMJ appliance?**

CHERYL: I used to get a lot of fatigue when I was on the regular Requip and that's why I switched to the XL. So I don't seem to get that as much anymore.

> **Caller 5: Is your concentration and memory getting better?**

CHERYL: I'm thinking more quickly than I was before; I'm speaking more quickly. I think they're starting to make more sense.

TMJ and Parkinson's Disease

I'm feeling more confident, definitely more confident. I'm feeling more like I can do things that I wouldn't undertake before; I can tackle more problems and I can take on more. I'm able to do more than I was before. I know a lot of people struggle with depression. I don't get depressed; I've never had that issue. I don't have hallucinations, depression, any of those things so I can't speak to any of those cognitive issues.

> **Caller 5: Have you talked to any of the people that have used the retainers over the long-term?**

CHERYL: I asked my dentist that question. He said the longest patient he's has treatment has been one year. I personally know one person who has used the appliance for seven months. He is the guy who told me he's a thousand times better. I love that number. When he said that - a thousand times - mostly people say "I'm a hundred percent better," he said, "I'm a thousand times better." I

TMJ and Parkinson's Disease

thought that was great. Then he said, "Cheryl, I'm symptom free, I'm completely normal" quote unquote. Those were his direct words to me. He looks like a real sharp guy, he's probably in his early 50s and he's right on top of things. He runs two businesses, he's got a pretty wife; he's got his life back. I did not ask him if he's med-free, and I wish I had, because I don't know that. But I did read a letter from him saying that he had reduced his meds, but I don't know if he's actually med-free or not.

Caller 5: So you're also doing chiropractic adjustments like once a week?

CHERYL: Yes. Fifteen sessions were included in the fee. The chiropractor I saw was <u>SOT certified</u>. He came to the dentist's office twice a week.

Caller 6: Did you ever previously experience any symptoms that would indicate a Temporo-mandibular condition to begin with?

TMJ and Parkinson's Disease

CHERYL: No, and that's what really concerned me because you have to answer a series of question and I was like, not applicable, not applicable, not applicable.

Caller 6: Did you ever have any pain in your mouth, in your jaw?

CHERYL: None at all. I never heard my jaw popping. I never had headaches. I never had whatever all those things that were on that list. I just couldn't answer yes to any of them and then that really scared me because I was like, "My God I don't even have any of these things, what am I doing here?"

Caller 6: This doesn't surprise me because what limited knowledge I have about the acupuncture meridians, the large intestine channel is, I would think the gateway into it is in your jaw and from some of the experience I've had in the past I think that large intestine channel that runs down your arm is actually deeply

TMJ and Parkinson's Disease

interrupted in a Parkinson's condition. I'm just wondering if by opening up this joint if you're actually opening up that large intestine channel too.

CHERYL: He's explained it to me three times, the mechanics of this and I can talk very minimally about it. It's kind of like, "Frankly my dear, I don't give a damn." I just want to see the result. So I don't care how the car runs, I just want it to run. I know that there are a lot of people who are technically-minded and that it has to make sense to them before they try it and from what you're talking about, it is just a little bit beyond me in scope. I have heard it opens up airways and it stops blockages in the Carotid artery which restricts the blood flow going to your brain. So it does make sense to technical people once they understand the mechanics behind it.

Caller 6: I think this is really curious because you're what I would call an

TMJ and Parkinson's Disease

early on-set patient and I have always postulated that the early on-setters tend to be people that were born with the condition or they're pre-dispositioned to the condition from environmental toxicity exposure of one sort or another and like you say who knows? You can think this thing from here to eternity and get a million different answers.

CHERYL: There is no history of Parkinson's in my family, more men than women get it. People who are older are more likely to have it than younger people. I just don't fall into any of the statistics, not really. The doctor told me that it was most likely environmental - like you're saying - and that a trauma to the body would have triggered it. The trauma to my body was giving birth to my child. He said it could be a car crash or something like that. It was lying dormant and the trauma to the body just triggered it. He said it would have come out

TMJ and Parkinson's Disease

eventually and that I probably had it for years. It was one year after the birth of my child when I started actually saying that something was wrong. I had known it for a couple of months afterwards but you don't know if it's the pregnancy with your first child. You just don't know what your body's doing. It's healing after the birth. It is adjusting. Then, different things start happening. You just keep thinking that it will go away and it doesn't. It starts getting worse and then after a year's time you have to pay attention to it. That's probably what triggered it for me.

Caller 7: Are you a single parent?

CHERYL: I'm a single parent.

Caller 7: I just wondered if that was a situation where you had to convince your partner that this is something that could be profitable.

CHERYL: It is definitely profitable as far as your health goes. Once you get your health back then everything else will flow

© *Parkinsons Recovery*   42

back together in your family I'm sure. It just makes things that much easier. Quite frankly it's cheaper than cost of my medicine and cost of doctor visits and the future cost of all this. I don't know where this is going. I don't know that I'm going to be med-free. I don't know if any of that's going to happen. I just know I'm able to do more. I'm feeling better. I'm seeing a reversal of my symptoms. I'm able to do things that I couldn't do and it just comes onto you. It's not like you try to do something that you couldn't do before. All of the sudden you start doing it.

Caller 7: Like being able to pull your pants up. When you said that, I was like, 'Right on girlfriend!' I know what you're saying. Do you exercise at all with your Parkinson's, are there other things you do to compliment what you're doing with the retainer?

CHERYL: I've never exercised in my life. I

know I should, everybody tells me, my girlfriends, everybody gets on me. I'm five foot four and I'm 120 pounds and I'm not out of shape.

Caller 7: Did you notice that you had Parkinson's on one side of your body and not on the other?

CHERYL: It started on my left side, absolutely and luckily I'm right-handed because I know that some people are right-handed and it started on their right side.

Caller 7: Did you ever get a cranial-sacral head massage?

CHERYL: No I haven't.

Caller 7: I did that once and I've done the Bowen Therapy and that helps but it only lasts for about a day to two days. The neat thing about the retainer is it'll move your jaw and it'll keep it open whereas the massage has probably opened up the areas for

© *Parkinsons Recovery*

TMJ and Parkinson's Disease

better blood flow but it doesn't stay open.

CHERYL: I've tried the hyperbaric chamber and that put more oxygen into my brain, compressed oxygen that you're sitting in a chamber and so it opens up your lungs and it opens up the oxygen into your brain and that seems to help but not even for a day; I'd say maybe for a couple of hours. Otherwise I haven't found any therapy that's really as compelling as this. It's a process, I'm not 100%. I'm not Parkinson's-free, I still need my medication but I feel so much better. Things are just coming back to me now.

Caller 7: You speak very well. I can tell because I know that feeling of when you're speaking and then you can't quite get the words like you want to, and you don't, you're not there, you're beyond that, you're back to normal speaking which is great to hear; it's convincing just listening to

you talk.

CHERYL: *Thank you so much. I couldn't have sustained a conversation this long and my voice would have been faded by now.*

Caller 7: Were you ever tested for heavy metals?

CHERYL: *Yes I did, I did the Wilson's test. I didn't have heavy mercury, I didn't have copper, I didn't have whatever else they tested for. I just remember those two in particular that weren't an issue.*

Caller 7: I guess the interesting thing about Parkinson's is that everybody's so different.

CHERYL: *I know; they call it the Designer's Disease. I don't really get the tremors so much. A lot of people have the shakes or the toe rolling hand motion, I don't get any of that stuff, not unless I'm really stressed out or nervous about something, then I'll start tremoring or if*

TMJ and Parkinson's Disease

I'm confronted with something that I don't want to be confronted with, then the shakes come in but on a whole I don't really get the tremors.

I've noticed that my balance is probably my biggest problem. But let me tell you, since my balance is improving my back doesn't hurt, and my feet had calluses on them because I was trying to compensate in keeping myself balanced in inappropriate ways. I developed these horrible calluses on my feet that I never had before and my calluses are going away. Just one correction corrects so many other things down the line, it's amazing.

Another thing that just happened this morning, they sound like such little things but they're huge in my world – I was able to squat down and just pet my cat without falling over. That just never happens, I always have to hold onto something or I would fall over. I did it for a few minutes.

TMJ and Parkinson's Disease

I could have stayed down there longer. It was amazing to me.

I was just like, wow, and so many things happen that I realize that I couldn't do and so many things happen to me that somebody else points out to me that they've realized that I couldn't do that, I didn't even realize that I couldn't do, so it's really fun to watch the whole thing unfold. It just happened so naturally, I just bent down and started petting my cat and I didn't fall over and then you consciously think, hey, I'm not falling over. You know, you don't consciously think, I'm going to bend down and I better hold onto something, it's interesting the way it works; it just happens so naturally it's unbelievable.

Caller 7: The symptoms you listed ... I was just so amazed ... 'That's me to a tee!' Even getting out of bed has only gotten worse in the last month and a half. I did too much in the last month and it caught up with me and it just

TMJ and Parkinson's Disease

made my Parkinson's symptoms escalate and nothing you can do about it then. You just have to rest and relax and listen to a show like this and get encouraged to think, 'Gosh, maybe there is something I can do to help reverse the symptoms instead of saying, 'Well, I put myself in this worse situation how is it going to remedy itself?' But I exercise a lot and I really know that helps me a lot. When I don't walk enough I can feel it the next day. But I'm so excited to think about something that could open up the flow of whatever, because I can see the blood not flowing in my legs and my hands. My hands are always cold. My feet are always cold and swollen.

CHERYL: The swelling in my feet has gone away. I had the same thing.

Caller 7: I know it's hard when there's not clinical research and proof. I've

TMJ and Parkinson's Disease

been doing Intravenous I.V. of glutathione and that's helped but it only helps for like three days. But I can't afford to do it three times a week because it's expensive and I think what you're doing with the mouth is like fixing what's causing the problem which is great because then the dopamine cells should be able to make their dopamine when they've got the blood flowing through there or whatever they need that wasn't coming in before, seems to make sense to me, anyway. How old are you?

CHERYL: I'm 52. I've had this for 10 years; I started noticing the symptoms when I was 42.

Caller 7: I'll be 58 this year and I started when I was 53. I've had it five years so I was sort of in that same category. The only difference is my mother had Parkinson's, but she had

TMJ and Parkinson's Disease

it very late in life. I was in a car accident before my Parkinson's symptoms started to show up which is like they say, the trauma and then it erupts.

CHERYL: *It is interesting you got yours after the car accident.*

Caller 7: Which I'm thinking maybe something got knocked out of place. It could be; I mean it was not a horrific accident, it was like a 30-mile an hour type, they ran a red light but I still got knocked around. So anyway I'm excited to try this, I think it could definitely be a help.

CHERYL: *I know it can be a help. I know it will; especially because you sound a lot like me. You sound like you're just experiencing a lot of things that I was experiencing. I don't see why you can't experience the wellness that I'm experiencing.*

Caller 8: How long does the process take from the time you initially go to the dentist to when you get the appliance?

CHERYL: I would say it would take you a maximum of three weeks before you could actually get your appliance from start to finish and then you could start wearing your appliance within the first two and half, three weeks.

It seems too good to be true and that's what scared me about it the most. It was just too unbelievable and I know how crazy it must sound especially because there's no research on it and there's no studies and there's never going to be any studies and your doctor's going to tell you not to do it and all your friends are going to tell you you're crazy.

I really hope I can make a difference in somebody else's life. If I've reached out and just got one more person, that's another starfish that gets thrown back in the ocean.

TMJ and Parkinson's Disease

How to Hear Cheryl on Parkinsons Recovery Radio

Visit http://www.blogtalkradio.com/parkinsons-recovery and scroll back to find the show that aired October 21, 2010 featuring Cheryl as my guest.

About Cheryl Epstein:

I was born a New Yorker. I lived on Long Island until I was 19. In 1984 I moved to Long Beach, CA where I still am today. I graduated from Long Beach State University with a BA in Sociology. I worked in the car business for 20 years.

I started seeing my first symptoms of Parkinson's October of 2000. I was diagnosed January, 2002. I gave birth to my second child Jan 2003. Luckily, I hadn't started medication yet. I nursed my son for 18 months until July 2004 when I was so sick from the symptoms of Parkinson's I had to stop nursing, and I began taking Parkinson's medication. Today I am a proud stay-at-home-mother of Sophie,

TMJ and Parkinson's Disease

age 11 and Luke age 8.

I am active in the kids' schools with PTA and serving on the School Site Council. I am also active with The League of Women Voters. I am in charge of health, education and safety. I am chief cook and bottle washer, taxi, friend, mother, daughter, sister, and woman in charge of my life. I also have two cats, both 21 years old, a garden, places to go, things to do, and people to see. I have a lot to take care of; I don't have time for Parkinson's. Thank you for listening to my story. You can contact me through my email at: mailto:sophieskutch@aol.com